Copyright © 2022 by Shannon Sánchez

SANCHEZ PUBLISHING INC.

All Rights Reserved.

Dedication

This book is dedicated to three very special and strong women in my life – my Mother, Nancy Selsor, my Granny, Esther Kueneke, and my Grandmother, Lucille Selsor. I owe all of my accomplishments to you. Thank you for showing and teaching me strength, determination, overcoming adversity, what it means to serve and befriend everyone around me, the importance of laughter, a sense of humor, and living life to the fullest. You will always be in my heart, and your legacy will live on for generations to come. I love you and thank you!

Shannon – Shan – Shanny

Forward

Shannon Sánchez effectively shares her personal experience of living with Polycystic Ovarian Syndrome (PCOS). She is vulnerable, engaging, and offers valuable advice to women who have PCOS and other health concerns. She offers resources and practical suggestions that are useful for women with PCOS and will assist them in navigating the health care system. Shannon's insights will give hope to women who have struggled with PCOS from an early age and will give hope to mothers with daughters who have PCOS. Be sure to use her workbook that accompanies this autobiography, *Kick PCOS to the Curb – The PCOS Lifestyle Workbook.*

Today, health care providers have made advancements in the diagnosis of PCOS. This book will be a benefit to them as a resource for their patients learning how to live with this complex syndrome.

Sister Marie Paul Lockerd, RSM, DO

www.rsmofalma.org

Table of Contents

Preface

It shouldn't be a surprise that a growing number of women in the United States experience menstrual problems. Some recent studies suggest that up to a third of American women today struggle with reproductive issues in their childbearing years ranging from irregular periods (me), PMS (me), unbalanced hormones (me), polycystic ovarian syndrome (me again), infertility, endometriosis, and others. *What's happening to us? Why are these illnesses increasing among women in the US (and in other developed countries of the world)? Why are there so many mothers and daughters struggling to understand their cycles despite advances in science and understanding of the human body?* Lifestyle, lifestyle, lifestyle.

I'm not a doctor. I do have a story to tell, though, that may help you or someone you know more fully understand these real struggles that affect millions of women, girls, and their families. It took me 25 years to gain a basic understanding of my unique body, cycle, and fertility, with many hurdles to overcome along the way. If sharing my journey can help even just one girl avoid these same struggles to some degree, writing this book is well worth it to me.

I'm a working mother of four young children ages seven, six, five, and four. My husband and I know time constraints and busy schedules all too well. I want this book to be a quick and easy read for you with helpful information and ideas that have helped me in my journey of overcoming PCOS – polycystic ovarian syndrome. Because we're talking all things menstruation, I should warn you of "TMI" at times.

I have three daughters and one son, but not in that order – girl, boy, girl, girl. That's a lot of estrogen coming my way in the near future! I think about the past 25 years of my life – since that dreaded day I started my period – and what I do as a mother now to hopefully avoid my daughters having similar issues as me when they reach puberty. So I'm writing this book to help women struggling with their cycle and hormones, husbands and fathers wanting to invest in their wives' and daughters' health to better support them, doctors and medical students, especially gynecologists and endocrinologists, who want to be able to better understand their patients with chronic illnesses, and of course mothers like me who want to help their daughters embrace the beauty of being a woman by learning more about their unique cycle and hormone needs.

I don't fault anyone for my struggles over the years with PCOS – surely not God, not my amazingly wonderful parents. Not even my doctors (and I've seen a lot of them), although I have wondered how much some of them have kept up on current research. Maybe I should fault genes? For sure society and the way we live today. And for sure our broken "health" care system, or as YouTube Doctor Sten Ekberg more appropriately calls it, "sick" care system (meaning there's little-to-no focus on being healthy and proactive in our current system – it's mostly reactive care after we've already gotten sick).

I also wasn't taught about my cycle in school, at least nothing beyond the general *"the average woman has a 28 day cycle and ovulates around day 14"*. Just a few years into getting my period I remember thinking maybe I was part woman part alien or something, because there didn't seem to be anything "normal" or "average" about my cycle. I remember feeling alone and different. I remember wearing a swimsuit one summer in high school and having a male friend tell me I had really hairy boobs – not something a young, impressionable girl wants to hear, *ever*! Talk about feeling embarrassed.

Today I'm 38 and I still have black hairs that grow on my right breast, along with on other unwanted parts of my body! (more about all that later) That's ok. God and my family have always loved me just the way I am. Read on to know what I know now, what I wish I had known years ago, and how I've overcome adversities from PCOS.

Introduction

It's been about 25 years since I started my period. If I had known at that moment that it would take 25 years to gain a basic understanding of my body and cycle I might have considered ripping my ovaries out right then and there. I got the basic gist of menstruation in middle school – I have this cycle thing, there's blood, boys don't have one, I could get pregnant, use a tampon or pad to catch the blood – that's about all I recall understanding at the time – pretty typical for a pre-teen girl. I remember doctors asking during normal check-ups when I had started my last period. (And they still focus mostly on the period, at least in my experience, even though *when a woman or girl last ovulated* would be a better question to ask at times, according to what I've learned. I suspect that more focus is given to the period simply because it's harder to detect ovulation.) I would usually give them incorrect dates or tell them I didn't remember. No one really told me to keep track.

Months in between periods didn't make it easier to remember either. I didn't know what a hormone was or how euphorically pleasant or horrendously wretched they could make my life. *Xeno—estro—andro—testo—WHAT*?! (xenoestrogens, estrogens, androgens, testosterone) Maybe (a very little maybe) sometime in high school I was taught estrogen and progesterone = girl; testosterone = boy, although truthfully I don't ever remember being fully taught that by anyone except YouTube in college.

I'm getting ahead of myself. I'll go back to the hormonal teenager in chapter 1. Who am I today in a nutshell?

Proud wife of nine years. Mother to my four beautiful angelitos (little angels in Spanish) – Olivia, Juan Pablo, Clarita, y Carolina. We are a bilingual, multicultural familia. My husband,

Marco, is from México. I have a Bachelor's degree in Spanish, a Master's degree in teaching, and an educational specialist degree in curriculum and instruction. I have visited a dozen different countries during countless international trips for school, medical mission work as an interpreter, chaperoning high school students, and for vacation. Marco and I speak Spanish to our kids at home. The older three are fully bilingual for their age and Carolina is well on her way at four-years-old. We are known in the neighborhood as the crazy, loud Spanish-speaking family. I don't try to hide it; I embrace it. We have a lot of crazy wrapped in a lot more love.

I'm the oldest of five children. I have a younger sister and three younger brothers. I have the best parents a child could ask for. My dad is a deacon in our local Catholic Church and Chief Mission Integration Officer for Catholic Charities (also a retired senior director from AT&T), and my mom is a well-respected retired Catholic school teacher in our community. I grew up in Kimmswick, Missouri, a small, historic town located on the Mississippi River south of St. Louis.

I'm a proud Catholic Christian. I live for God. I pray multiple times a day, starting with a decade of the Rosary on my way to work every morning. My kids and I especially pray to our Blessed Mother and ask for her intercession to our daily prayers, just like my parents used to do with my siblings and me when we were younger. That is how I learned to pray. I do what I can to serve and befriend all of God's people whom I encounter. I have a big imagination. I love working with people, sharing ideas, and I love everything about teaching. I love that Jesus was known as the Master Teacher and I try to be like Him.

During my fifteen years so far working in education I have served in Catholic and public schools as a high school teacher, elementary principal, and curriculum, instruction, and academic programs director for preschool through high school.

Let's talk hormones, acne, yeast infections, panic attacks – you name it, I've had it when it comes to hormone problems. I sincerely hope this book helps you, even if just learning a few things to try for you or for a loved one (or if you are a doctor, for one of your patients). If it helps you, please share the book with others who may need it. I always reference Mother Theresa's famous quote when teaching or sharing information with others – "I can do things you cannot; you can do things I cannot; **together** we can do great things." I'm honored to share my journey with you.

Chapter 1

TEENAGE YEARS WITH PCOS

I've heard lots of people say they would never want to relive their teenage years – I'm with you! I have many great memories from being a teenager, but also many that I would much rather forget. Now I know the memories I would rather forget are mostly tied to PCOS, directly or indirectly. When I think of those years, I think of acne, Accutane, Minocycline, Tetracycline, extreme red faces, countless trips to the dermatologist. (It's amazing that I made it through all those appointments without ever ripping that devilish silver metal pimple popper instrument out of the doctor's hands and throwing it at him!) I think of crying, sobbing sometimes for no reason, anxiety, stomach—chin—boob, and—upper lip black hairs (and to make it worse, I'm a blonde), double period months, three months without a period, too much vaginal discharge (mucus, bacterial, yeast – gross!)

I remember hearing girls in school talk about how many days apart their periods were. I remember thinking (but never saying out loud), *Something must be wrong with me cause I never know when my next period will be.* I definitely had no clue when I was ovulating, and, again, I don't remember ever being asked questions or talking about ovulation. Everything was about the period. I remember being told that my irregular periods were probably due to being athletic, although looking back, I don't think that was my case because I only played one sport at a time and never year round, so I wasn't overly athletic. I don't fault those doctors for getting me "wrong", not completely at least. I know there's a ton more research available today and a greater focus on PCOS and other reproductive illnesses (more focus because they're more prevalent today due to our lifestyle). But I do think more could have been done – more questions asked, more conversation, more time and education for my mom and me during those visits.

Looking back, I wish my doctors would have explored my unique conditions more thoroughly. I was a confused, clueless, emotional teenager with tiny ovarian cysts wreaking emotional and physical havoc on my body. And nobody knew it. It would take me 25 years exactly to figure out how to get them under control.

My diet wasn't helping AT ALL. Little was known back then about just how much diet influences a woman's cycle. Actually, what largely determines our cycle and hormones is our gut bacteria (also known as gut flora or microbiome). When our gut bacteria is unbalanced (too much bad bacteria and not enough good bacteria), disease is inevitable. Today's use of preservatives, antibiotics (given to animals we eat), and the methods used to process our food is not natural and introduces all kinds of chemicals into our bodies.

I have come to understand and believe wholeheartedly that *you are what you eat* is a profound truth that isn't taken seriously enough by many people. And our DNA is suffering more and more with each new generation of nugget and pizza-eating munchkins whose parents hope (and think) that their processed food can just be supplemented with vitamins. (But it doesn't work that way.)

Now let's talk about stress – When I was 15 I started working in the kitchen of a local resident's center preparing meals for the elderly. Seven hours of school, two hours of track practice (winter and spring), three hours of work, then home to do usually around five hours of homework = not enough sleep and way too much stress (cortisol hormone) for a young teenage girl. But I was never taught about cortisol – never heard of it til my 30's. (Pay close attention to how much I talk about cortisol throughout my journey.)

I transferred to a new high school my junior year, going from an all-girls Catholic city school to a co-ed Catholic country school. I don't know the exact impact that change of schools had on my hormones and cycle, except for making me somewhat boy-crazy. I do believe my junior and senior years were less stressful as I didn't have to study as much to get good grades at my new school. And I believe that had a positive impact on my cortisol levels. I was extremely self-conscious, though. Always worried about what others were thinking of me.

Being overly self-conscious is such an exhausting burden that I don't wish for anyone – more cortisol, yay. I think some of it was due to personality and genes – I am a self-criticizing and people-pleasing INFJ perfectionist through-and-through. Maybe some stress (cortisol) from being the oldest of my siblings, which automatically brings added, and often times unwanted, attention, especially for an introvert. I was "the guinea pig" of my parents' five kids, as they say. Every family has one. But in addition to genes, oldest-child syndrome, and normal (millennial) teenage selfishness assuming the whole world was thinking about "me", without a doubt, a lot of my self-consciousness came from the PCOS hormonal rollercoaster.

Don't get me wrong, I have some amazing memories from those years. I wasn't miserable 24/7. From the outside I'm sure I looked like a pretty normal teen. My hormones were just out of control due to the normal process of fertility making too many small egg sacks (follicles) and none of them coming to the point of ovulation, thus throwing off the normal hormonal ebb and flow. And that's PCOS in a nutshell.

Things would get way worse before they got better. I graduated high school and went on taking classes towards an associate's degree at a local community college. After I turned 19 I started randomly breaking out in horrendously itchy hives all over my body. I never knew when they would come on or how long they would last. Sometimes I would be in a swimming pool,

sometimes in a store, sometimes watching tv. I remember curling
up in a ball and wrapping myself in a heavy blanket in an attempt
to not feel the itchiness as much. When the hives would move to
my hands and feet, that was the worst! I would scratch until my
skin bled. My mom took me to see my primary care doctor and I
was referred to an allergist. I was told to keep a journal to track
what I ate and what I was doing leading up to each hives
breakout. I did. For months. Nothing made sense. There were no
obvious patterns. My asthma was getting worse too. I had
experienced athletic-induced asthma as a kid and used albuterol
as necessary, but once the hives came on at 19 I found myself
needing my inhaler more and more as well. *What was going on
with me?!*

Cats and dogs.

Excuse me?? That was our reaction when we were told after
my prickly needle allergy test results came back that I was mildly
allergic to dogs and highly allergic to cats. But I had practically
lived in a zoo my entire life up to that point – seriously, cats,
dogs, rabbits (started out with three and rather quickly turned into
21), a bird, fish, hermit crabs, iguanas, horses and chickens at my
grandparents' farm – you name it we had it. I had never had
issues with animals or allergies, so the test had to be wrong.

"Not so", said the doctor. I remember him using a "snap of
fingers" to explain just how quickly someone's allergies could
change. I remember feeling *extra* lucky when he then explained
in a matter-of-fact way that while childhood allergies often times
go away, allergies that come on as an adult can and often times
do last a lifetime.

Sheesh. Ok so irregular periods, acne, rosacea, asthma, and
now severe allergies to cats and dogs that turn into full body
hives. But again, all things considered, I seemed like a pretty
normal, healthy young adult. I thought I was healthy, at least. I
exercised a lot. I had a normal weight. I didn't eat very well but I
took vitamins. I remember thinking, *Who eats the recommended*

amount of fruits and vegetables today anyway?? That's what *vitamins are for.* If only I had known better.

Chapter 2
THE ROARING 20'S WITH PCOS

By 20-years-old I had finished my associate's degree and had transferred to a four-year university about 30 minutes from home. I was granted work study hours to help pay for tuition. My parents joked that they found out I was allergic to cats and dogs so they got rid of me instead of the pets – *haha, funny*. Really I decided to move out because my work study hours and class schedule had me opening the campus gym at 5:30 in the morning, classes scattered throughout the day, and often times closing the gym at midnight. Spending hours (and gas money that I didn't have) commuting back-and-forth every day and literally taking long naps and breaks in my car wasn't ideal. So I took out a student loan to live in the apartments on campus.

I was officially on my own. Was I ready to be on my own? Heck no. But there was no convincing me otherwise. For a 20-year-old I was a hard worker, independent, and extremely determined. I had been working since 15 so I was already pretty accustomed to earning money and paying bills.

Side note – my hives continued even after moving into a no animal policy apartment. After dabbling with a few allergy medicines that didn't work for me (Allegra, Claritin, Benadryl), I found Zyrtec. Despite never being around cats and dogs anymore, my hives continued. I told this to my doctors over the next several years and they just said to keep taking the Zyrtec because I was probably sensitive to histamine and Zyrtec is antihistamine. *Okay?* So I did, every day, 20 mg, for what would turn into 16 years. What would happen if I forgot? The hives would come back with a vengeance. Literally I couldn't even walk down the street on a hot summer day without getting itchy if I had forgotten to take my Zyrtec.

When I was 21 I got Mono – that wasn't fun. I was so fatigued for months. Add to that work, paying bills, all the normal *living on your own responsibilities*, keeping up with my studies. What does that spell? Too much cortisol!

Fast forward another year – I was 22 and finishing my last few courses towards a Bachelor's degree in Spanish at a university in Argentina. I had done a lot of international traveling for my Bachelor's degree – traveling through Spain, working in Peru several times as a medical interpreter for a mission organization, and finishing courses in Argentina. When finished, I decided to accept an opportunity to teach high school Spanish where I had graduated high school just four years before. *Could I be a teacher?* My mom was a Catholic elementary school teacher. I thought (very foolishly), *teaching can't be that hard.*

I was so young that I sometimes got mistaken for being a student. "Students can't use the copy machine, honey", I remember a nice lady in the main office telling me once. I smiled and told her I was a teacher.

My first year of teaching was every bit what they say first year teaching is – really hard!!! On top of being a short 22-year-old female teaching mostly students who were taller than me without ever having completed a single teaching course in college, I was sick *constantly*. The Urgent Care doctors closest to my apartment came to know me really well that year. In fact, I was prescribed *five* Z-pack antibiotics within my first year of teaching for sinus infections – no joke. That was the 2006-2007 school year, when we were still popping antibiotics like candy. I used to think the sinus infections were a combination of mold in the old school building plus students sharing all sorts of viruses with me I had never contracted before. Hindsight 2020, why had I not gotten sick so often just four years prior when I was a student in the same building? Answer – *stress – cortisol*. Much more on stress later and how it has affected my hormones and cycle.

I now know all those antibiotics were killing good bacteria in my stomach and intestines on top of killing all the junk in my sinuses. Of course back then, I didn't have a clue about the massive destruction going on in my digestive system and the subsequent brain inflammation – I just wanted all the green junk out of my nose and ears so I could sleep. Speaking of sleep – I don't remember having issues getting enough z's when I was a kid, but I definitely had become a poor sleeper as I got older. During my third year of teaching at age 25 I had a tonsillectomy. I remember my ENT saying that when he started cutting into my tonsils they exploded like a kid squeezing a tube of tooth paste. Um, gross. Sleep did not get any better after that. More on sleep later.

During one of my medical mission trips to the third world country of Peru, South America, I was the interpreter for a gynecologist. During one of our breaks I started telling her about my irregular periods. She recommended I come see her when we got back to St. Louis. I did, and she put me on the pill, saying that it would help my hormones even out. What a crock of BS that was! But again, I didn't know better. She was a highly educated, experienced, and confident professional. I was a young, impressionable girl in my mid 20's who didn't know anything about my body. So I listened to her.

I really didn't have much time to think about my health either. By that time I was working four jobs to pay for a Master's degree out of pocket. No joke, I was teaching high school full-time during the day, Monday and Wednesday evenings I was teaching ESL classes to immigrant families in St. Louis who had been transferred from somewhere around the world, I was teaching fitness classes (pilates, yoga, and cycling) Thursday evenings and Saturday mornings, and bar-tending Friday and Saturday nights.

Sheesh. Just typing that out made me tired. But that was my life. I made those decisions. In order to keep teaching I needed to obtain certification, and the only difference between my certification and a Master's in teaching was 12 credit hours plus a thesis, so I decided to keep at it.

You know what all that spells? More *stress – cortisol*. Yep. I can't imagine how much of it I had in my body during those years, especially the few years when I was on the pill. I, like many girls, did not have a good experience on the pill. Lots of anxiety, acne, more anxiety, and more acne. But I was having "regular" periods, sooooo?

I say "regular" because I don't believe there's anything regular about pumping a ton of synthetic hormones into a girl's body (what I knew back then versus what I know now). For one thing, every person has a unique, delicate hormone level balance and physiology. So the pill is essentially a one-size-fits-all approach. Everyone is different. Some girls are prone to having higher levels of androgens (male hormone). Some have lower levels of androgens. Some are extra sensitive to estrogens and the many foods and chemicals that our bodies "read" as estrogen. Some are low in progesterone. You get the idea. And our hormones are always changing. So basically without any attempt whatsoever to understand my unique hormone levels and physiology, an experienced, professional doctor just had me start popping daily hormone bombs like candy. I'm sure she got paid big bucks from big pharma while I got acne and anxiety.

Secondly, the pill, and all contraceptives used as medicine, are really just band aids used to subside annoying symptoms that come from much deeper issues. Birth control is not a cure for any medical condition. It was created to allow men and women to have sex without making a baby. I truly believe the creation of the pill has been one of the greatest downfalls of our nation and world in modern history, directly and indirectly leading to all kinds of destruction – breakdown of marriage and family values, increased physical and mental health issues among women, increased pregnancies outside of marriage and single mothers, and more.

Back to my 20's. I went off the pill after a few years. I was told by that doctor that for some women being on the pill for a while can somehow magically "kick start" their hormones into gear. That did not happen for me. (I wonder if it actually happens for some women?) I went to see an endocrinologist about my increasingly irregular periods. Here's a recap of how that appointment went:

Doctor   *You have irregular periods?*

Me   *Yes, ever since I started my period.*

Doctor   *You may have PCOS – polycystic ovarian syndrome. It's little cysts that grow on a woman's ovaries. About 10% of women have it.*

Me   *Okay*

Doctor   *Let's do an ultrasound to check for them.*

Me   *Okay* (We go to the ultrasound room.)

Doctor   *Yep, what do ya know, there they are.* (Points out all the tiny pearl-looking-things around my ovaries.)

Okay, okay, there was a little more to the conversation, but not much. *When was your last period? How far apart are they typically? Anything you know of that makes them worse?* But for the most part it was *"Hey you have PCOS. Ok here's the bill. Thanks for coming in!"*

I didn't know what to ask, so I didn't ask anything. And I was told nothing. Nothing! Not what causes it. Not what cures it. Not how it was likely impacting my body. Not how to manage it. NOOOOTHING!

So the only difference that appointment made was to my health insurance bill that month and to future health questionnaires where I started ignorantly writing down PCOS in the section on known medical conditions. Despite switching gynecologists and primary care doctors later in my 20's, believe it or not it would still be another 10 years before I would come to understand PCOS and my unique cycle.

Chapter 3

BALANCE IN MY 30'S

MARRIAGE, KIDS, WORK, MARRIAGE, KIDS, WORK WITH PCOS

I met my husband on CatholicMatch.com when I was 28. He was 39 and living in Beaumont, Texas on a work visa at the time. Married at 29, first child at 30, and in the blink of an eye I was 34, married with four kids ages 3, 2, 1, and newborn (insert big yawn and even bigger coffee mug). Not to mention I was a new elementary school principal (preschool, elementary, and middle school). With my second and third children (back-to-back July babies), I really didn't even have maternity leave. It was like the kids popped out, I said *nice to meet you, honey* (really it was *mucho gusto, cariño*), and I was back in the office within a few days preparing things for the new school year. I actually hired a teacher from my hospital bed in July, 2015 waiting for Juan Pablo to make his debut.

I love working for the Catholic Church and for Catholic education. There are a lot of benefits like having the opportunity to go to Mass every day at work and receive the sacrament of Confession every week. The Eucharist and Confession are God's pathways (gifts) to each of us that help us stay close to Him and come to discover His plan for us. But I wish they would have had better maternity leave benefits when I was having my babies. To some degree, I knew what I was getting into when signing my contracts, but still. Anyway, I'm happy to report that I currently work in the education office of that same archdiocese as part of a great group of dedicated people working to make necessary changes that will even better support families within our communities moving forward.

Back to pregnancies. First of all, remember I never knew when I was going to get a period, much less when or even *if* I ever ovulated. Clearly I figured out that, yes, I did in fact ovulate. But when? No clue. I have talked to women who are actually able to sense and pin point the exact seconds that they ovulate. I'm happy for them. I think it's amazing that they are able to know and be in touch with their bodies that well. But in my case, that's in the category of someday being six feet tall – not gonna happen for me.

Something very interesting, considering my decades-long cycle struggles, was that I had very pleasant, enjoyable pregnancies. While I will never know the exact reasoning behind that, I suspect it was due to all the "feel good" hormones that typically accompany pregnancy. Considering I was practically prego for four years straight, I had a lot of "feel good" hormones during those years. After reading about the struggles of getting pregnant with PCOS (there's a lot more research available now than there was just a decade ago), I was baffled that I popped out four kids so fast with no issues. I was never even trying to get pregnant!

Months after my fourth baby was born in January, 2018, sometime after I stopped nursing, my body started to go haywire – like a different level of haywire I had never experienced before. It was bad. Of course my cycle was still irregular, still had acne and rosacea, still taking 20 mg of Zyrtec every day to keep hives at bay (cause I was still allergic to "cats and dogs" – insert eye roll). Despite the Zyrtec and tonsillectomy I was still getting frequent sinus infections, still had black hairs and all that jazz. But on top of *all* that, my anxiety and irritability were through the roof and I couldn't sleep. I was having these massive mood swing blow ups like a volcano that goes from dormant to spewing hot lava within seconds.

It makes me sad thinking of who bore the brunt of my anger during those years – my kids. My husband of course as well, but at least as a mature adult he was able to compartmentalize my issues and not take them personally. The good thing is that kids are resilient and I have explained to them, in ways they can understand, why I was like that back then so they don't feel guilty or like they were at fault for something.

Most days it felt like I was hanging on by a thread. Things were hard back in my 20's, but I was just responsible for me during those years, and I was in control of everything (control can be the evilest of demons, especially for a perfectionist – more on that later). It felt like I woke up one day, still suffering the same PCOS issues, and all the sudden balancing a marriage and four littles as well (aka not in control of anything anymore!). I loved my new little family more than anything. I knew each one of them was a precious gift from God. There was so much joy – giggles, smiles, milestones. But I couldn't fully embrace the joy with the silent war going on inside my body.

I went to see my regular gynecologist who had delivered three of my four babies (different gyno from the one in my 20's). I loved having her deliver my babies, but she, too, just wanted to put me on the pill – surprise, surprise. So I went to see two new gynecologists, including one who specialized in PCOS. That doctor recommended I start taking Myo Inositol and D-Chiro Inositol, compounds naturally found in fruits and fiber-rich foods that can positively affect insulin levels, which are often times problematic for women with PCOS (research the links between PCOS and metabolic syndrome). So I added those to my daily (expensive) intake of vitamins and supplements, which was probably up to around 15 different types at that point. My whole cabinet was filled with vitamin and supplement bottles. I was desperate and willing to try anything. But Inositol wasn't the answer either. I tried it for months and never noticed a difference. I also didn't feel like that doctor took me very seriously, maybe because my PCOS didn't include fertility issues. I felt like she was thinking, *Really, you're here for PCOS and you're skinny with four kids under the age of five?* (Most women with PCOS have weight issues, but a small percentage of women have "lean

PCOS".) I called once to follow up with her and never got a call back.

So I had gone to see gynecologists of three different health care networks in St. Louis. I was very prepared at each appointment, bringing lists of my symptoms, cycle dates, general medical history information like when my hives started, dates of my surgeries, medicines, and a list of vitamins/supplements I was taking. None of them panned out to be any help and I was growing more desperate by the day. Like there was always a time bomb inside me and I never knew when the next mental explosion (breakdown) would occur.

My sinus issues were so bad, and I couldn't afford to take off work constantly, especially as a school principal. I was again chalking up the green junk in my head to working in an old building. I went to see my primary care doctor and she recommended I start taking a nasal spray on top of the Zyrtec. I also got an air purifier for my office. I went to see a different ENT than the one who had performed my tonsillectomy back in my 20's. He said I had a massively crooked septum and recommended I have a septoplasty to correct it. I went to get a second opinion and it came back the same – I had between a 90-95% blockage on the left side of my nasal passage, which made sense because my left side always seemed more clogged than the right. So I had a septoplasty. I thought, *what's one more surgery?* Wisdom teeth, tonsillectomy, C-section (just with the first baby; luckily I was able to V-back with the other three), and now septoplasty. *Maybe this will be the cure? At least for my sinuses?*

All throughout my struggles I was praying like crazy. Besides my wonderfully supportive family, especially my husband and parents, praying to Mary gave me more comfort than anything. I would think of all she endured during her life as the Mother of Jesus, especially having to watch His suffering and death on the Cross, and it would give me comfort. I also used to think of my grandmother who had 12 children, my granny who raised three kids on her own while working full-time, my mom – full-time teacher with us five little kids and my dad often times having to travel for work, and the many women of the world suffering in unique ways to help me through another day.

But I knew that Jesus didn't want me to suffer. He is the Healer of all Healers. The Master Teacher and Master Physician. So I kept fighting, receiving Communion at Mass for strength, protection, and wisdom, and praying to find answers.

One morning in January, 2019 I hit a new low. I was on my way to a work-sponsored school event to watch some of our archdiocesan high school bands play. It was nothing to stress over. I was going there as a representative of my office to cheer on our performing choir and band students and teachers. But all of the sudden I found myself driving on the highway and not being able to catch my breath. It was really scary. I was driving on a busy highway during rush hour traffic and I couldn't breathe, like there was a ton of bricks laying on top of my chest or something.

I called my dad, who I often call when feeling overwhelmed, and I remember it being so hard to get words to actually come out of my mouth to explain to him what was going on. He helped me get in a better mindset and I entered the school building praying to God that the day would go by as fast as possible. *What was going on with me?* There was NOTHING I needed to be stressing over (*ha* – besides the whole full-time working married mom of four kids thing). But really, it wasn't like other work events where sometimes I would be the presenter running the show. I was just there for moral support for our teachers and students. Now *I* was needing moral support to be able to give *them* moral support!

I remember being so overly self-conscious that day, like the whole world knew what was going on in my head. It's the weirdest thing to try and explain, but that entire morning I would open my mouth, even to just greet someone and words would not come out easily. It was somewhat like the feeling of blowing up a balloon. I had to fill my lungs with enough air just to force the words, *Hi how are you?* to come out. I remember thinking, *What is wrong with me?! This day is supposed to be all about them and all I can think about is myself!*, like my brain had somehow reverted back to puberty when all I cared about was me, myself, and I.

I survived the day, like every other day. My routine during those years had become work, feed kids, bathe kids, get kids to bed, get stuff ready for the next day (uniforms, lunches, etc.), then fanatically search the web on my cell phone for answers to what was wrong with me, since I still hadn't gotten answers from anywhere or anyone. Maybe I could find answers on YouTube.

My First Miracle -- The Creighton Model FertilityCare System & NaProTECHNOLOGY

Two recent "shifts" (I call them my own little miracles) have been monumental for me in finally getting a handle on my life and health during the last couple of years. And they are the two main reasons for writing this book. The first is thanks to Sister (Dr.) Marie Paul Lockerd DO (DO stands for Doctor of Osteopathic Medicine – an area of medicine that holistically studies the interrelated unity of all bodily systems).

I mentioned earlier that my dad is the Director of Catholic Charities for the Archdiocese of St. Louis. One day he introduced me to Dr. Sister Marie Paul Lockerd, a Catholic nun and physician of the Mercy Sisters of Alma order who ran the Archdiocesan *Rural Clinic* at the time, an RV clinic that travels to rural communities around the St. Louis area serving the poor with free health care. Among other areas, she specialized in women's fertility using NaProTECHNOLOGY (Natural Procreative Technology) and The Creighton Model FertilityCare System, a method created by Dr. Thomas Hilgers, Director of the Pope Paul VI Institute for the Study of Human Reproduction in Omaha,

Nebraska in the 1980's that teaches women how to track hormones and fertility with daily observations of their cervical mucus.

Umm, excuse me?? Cervical what?? Ok hang on, I have four little kids – four pregnancies, four deliveries and recoveries, I'm used to snot, poop, blood, vomit – you name it, I've done it when it comes to gross. But touching my own cervical mucus? Never heard of such a thing.

But apparently it's a thing. And she taught it to me. The next eight months were spent learning about my daily mucus and experimenting with hormone therapy based on characteristics of my mucus. She gave me a chart-like calendar with color-coded stickers that I would use to track characteristics of the mucus. In a nutshell, blood = period, dry or cakey mucus = non-fertile days, and slippery, stretchy mucus = fertile days. Pretty simple. Sometimes, especially in the beginning, I would take pictures of the mucus with my phone and text them to her to be sure I was coding correctly. She was very open to that, and I was very thankful for her always being available to me in that way. I would also document on the chart my mental and physical symptoms, although she taught me that figuring out my cervical mucus was key to deciding what hormone replacements I needed and during which days of my cycle.

I learned that the Creighton Model FertilityCare System, is the Catholic Natural Family Planning (NFP) charting system. NaProTECHNOLOGY is the medical intervention used when a women or couple requires more than the Creighton Model FertilityCare System.

> NaProTECHNOLOGY refers to Natural Procreative Technology, an approach to understanding women's reproductive health and regulating fertility by identifying and treating the underlying causes of problems—not simply placing a Band-Aid on them. Instead of treating symptoms, NaProTECHNOLOGY uses natural methods and restorative

surgery to treat diseases. It also pairs with the Creighton Model Fertility*Care*™ System, which actively engages a woman to track and manage her fertility. This scientific approach empowers a woman to be a key part of her Care Team and has been successful in treating a host of issues including infertility, endometriosis, menstrual pain, ovarian cysts, Polycystic Ovarian Syndrome, repetitive miscarriage, postpartum depression, hormonal abnormalities, bleeding disorders, chronic discharges, premenstrual syndrome, and premature birth. NaProTECHNOLOGY treats conditions cooperatively with the menstrual cycle and avoids the use of artificial hormones and devices to regulate fertility or control symptoms. NaProTECHNOLOGY's restorative approach to infertility costs less than IVF treatments and has proven highly successful in helping couples achieve healthy pregnancies. (Catholicmedicalcenter.org)

Back to my cycle. The tracking definitely validated PCOS. My cycle was a mess – all over the place, no pattern whatsoever. Some periods 70+ days apart, some 30 days apart. And I was hardly ever ovulating, which I learned can sometimes be a key factor in determining if a woman of childbearing years is healthy. Within a six month span I only had one fertile day, according to my mucus.

I know what you're thinking, I remember staring at my chart thinking it too. *Only one fertile day in six months?* How did I ever get pregnant four times in a row? I've asked myself that question too. Beyond the obvious biological answer, I believe wholeheartedly that God has a purpose for my kids, just as He has a purpose for everyone. Sadly still today, many people do not get the chance to discover their purpose. So reminding myself of that fact was, and still is today, key for me – my kids have a purpose and my #1 responsibility (vocation) as their parent on this earth is to help them figure out what that purpose is.

Back to hormones. Something interesting that became obvious as the months went on with my tracking was that I was generally feeling ok, even *good* at times, both during and right after my periods, but the further from a period I would get, the worse my physical and mental symptoms would become. And I would not have made those connections without someone teaching me how to track my mucus and symptoms. Thank you Dr. Sister Marie Paul! And thank you to everyone responsible for creating and promoting the Creighton Model FertilityCare System! I just wish I had known about it sooner.

Supposedly it was a focus of the Natural Family Planning (NFP) workshop my husband and I had to complete as part of our Catholic marriage preparation, but neither one of us remembers it. There was so much going on in our lives at that time, it's understandable why a topic briefly touched upon during a three hour workshop wouldn't stick in our brains. Plus by that time, after more than 15 years of struggling with PCOS, anyone who brought up the word "cycle" to me, automatically "lost me", because in my mind I didn't have a cycle. No one asked me any questions at that workshop. It was just a lot of information thrown at the participants – very little engagement. So I don't know how much I was actually paying attention.

Side note – why had none of my previous gynecologists ever mentioned any of this to me?!? Why were all those (wasted) appointments (wasted time, money, and energy) with specialists in female fertility and health just about my periods, pap smears, and *oh, birth control might help you since you have irregular periods.* REALLY!!?? That's what we're doing with women in this country despite all the advances in science and research today? Especially the research about the dangers of the pill?! This is unacceptable, and I'm sounding the alarm!!!

Ok back to my symptoms again. Like I said, they would all get worse the further away from a period I got. Physical – bloating (mid-section, hands, and face), extreme fatigue, acne, dry skin (especially lips and hands), night sweats, spotting dark discharge at times, and upper back and neck pain. The back of neck pain got so bad that I brought it up to my primary care doctor who sent me to physical therapy. That helped a little but not much. I did have a fabulous Catholic primary care doctor, Dr. Schmeidler, who had talked to me about trying anxiety medicine, but I didn't want to add any new medicines that might somehow skew the effects or results of what Dr. Sister Marie Paul and I were doing (more about Dr. Schmeidler later).

Mental symptoms – anxiety, irritability, anger, foggy brain (although when your brain isn't working it's hard to realize that your brain isn't working, so I realized that symptom much later than the others – in other words, I had foggy brain but didn't know at the time that I had foggy brain), and the dreadful blood and energy-sucking zombie, insomnia. Insomnia was 100% the worst of them all. Not being able to fall asleep or stay asleep is so incredibly exhausting – physically, mentally, and emotionally.

For a while I was trying every trick in the book to fall asleep and stay asleep because I had known a few people addicted to sleep meds, and I didn't want to add another issue to my already sky-high stack of issues. But Dr. Sister Marie Paul prescribed me a sleep aid and advised I take them with caution, just when I felt like I had gone days without a good night sleep and was desperate.

After we had gathered several months of data from using the Creighton Model, we started experimenting with hormone therapy. She warned me up front that it would take time to figure out exactly what I needed and when I needed it. She was also the one who explained to me how birth control is a one-size-fits-all approach. What we figured out for me is that I was extra sensitive to estrogen (probably why I didn't do well on the pill). She had me try taking low dose estrogen therapy (pills) a little after my period during my follicular phase (after period and before ovulation). I tried them during two different occasions (cycles) and both times resulted in tears, sensitivity, and moodiness.

Ok so estrogen wasn't my thing. Some women, especially women with irregular periods, are "estrogen dominant", meaning they have higher than normal levels of estrogen in their bodies. It can come from a variety of things, one culprit being "xenoestrogens". Remember the title – *Xeno-Estro-Andro-Testo WHAT?!* That was my response when first reading about this xenoestrogen phenomenon. Basically a lot of the junk we're exposed to today, thanks in part to being a first world country and having a lot of options (aka exposure to chemicals), is being "read" by our bodies as estrogen. Everything from certain types of plastics, synthetic chemicals in creams, make-up, deodorants, drier sheets, even really hard to avoid stuff like fire retardant chemicals in furniture are xenoestrogens.

So for instance, I put on deodorant. The deodorant I use isn't organic (side note – not everything that says organic on the label is actually organic). There's some dangerous chemicals in the deodorant (often times related to preservatives to extend the product's shelf life, which equals more money for the company). And my body "reads" those unnecessary chemicals as estrogen. My body is also producing its own estrogen. So now I have more estrogen than I need. And my high estrogen then throws off other hormone levels in my body. So estrogen therapy was *no bueno* for me.

Progesterone, on the other hand, was very much liked by my body. The tricky thing about progesterone was that starting to take those pills every month, if I hadn't yet ovulated, meant that I for sure wasn't going to ovulate during that cycle. In other words, there was still a chance I would ovulate, but starting to take the progesterone pills crushed that chance. The ideal scenario would be that I would ovulate, which would kick my body into gear making its own progesterone.

But no ovulation equaled no progesterone-production. And low progesterone for me equaled all those awful symptoms. So I needed to supplement (progesterone therapy). Within a couple days of taking bio-identical Prometrium (progesterone) pills, I would feel and look so much better. Most physical and mental symptoms would go away, or at least significantly diminish.

While the progesterone therapy was definitely helping to keep my symptoms at bay, my cycle wasn't getting any better. In other words, the progesterone was just a band aid – a very effective band aid, but it wasn't curing the root cause of my illness. So Dr. Sister Marie Paul suggested I try a light dose of an SSRI, selective serotonin reuptake inhibitor (anxiety and depression medicine). She had explained to me prior that the PCOS could very well be genetic.

I asked about genetic testing but decided that it wasn't worth the money or time. Let's say I find out that I do, in fact, have some gene mutation (like many people have) responsible for the PCOS. Currently there would be nothing I could do on top of everything else I'm already doing to fix it (eat healthy, exercise, get enough sleep, relax) – science is definitely moving in that direction but isn't quite there yet. Someday (my guess is sooner rather than later) we'll be able to walk into a doctor's office with mutated genes and come out with them magically fixed. But since that's currently not possibly, it doesn't really matter what my genes are. At least that's how I feel about it.

So I started to take 10 mg of Lexapro for anxiety on top of the progesterone as needed. It took a few months to start feeling a difference, but when I did it was pretty magical. The biggest improvement was in my overall mood. I felt that I could tolerate things easier – people, situations, life in general. She said I probably won't need it forever, maybe just to help me get through these stressful years working full-time with four babies, just to take the edge off.

A couple side notes about the Lexapro – I realized after about a year of my own trial and error that if I took the Lexapro earlier in the evening (as soon as I got home from work) that I would have less trouble falling asleep. For a while we increased the

Lexapro to 20 mg. That helped even more with my irritability, but it also left me "flat", emotionless, and fatigued. I am grateful for the Lexapro that helped me when I needed it. However, I have since learned from my rock star YouTube doctors that nutritional yeast and other supplements that balance our gut microbiome can be an effective, all-natural alternative to SSRI's (antidepressants). Recent meta-analysis studies are showing some alarming trends in people who have taken antidepressants long-term, including increased risks of heart attacks, strokes, and early death. *Umm, no thank you.* I have been slowly weaning my way off the Lexapro and leaning on Nutritional Yeast, as well as other lifestyle alterations that I talk about in the next chapter, and it's working for me.

Back to the Creighton Model. I love how much more I know about my body thanks to the Creighton Model. Who would have thought that knowing one's cervical mucus could teach so much. Only took me to age 36 to find it out! Why don't we teach this to girls in school?? Do you know how many mothers and daughters in my close circle of family and friends are on the pill simply because they have cycle issues?!?! The pill was never designed to be a fix for that! And this is not their fault! Again, I'm sounding the alarm to DOCTORS and BIG PHARMA to STOP prescribing and promoting the pill for reproductive issues!

So I had the progesterone to lean on for when my hormones seemed out of whack (when I knew, based on my mucus, that I hadn't ovulated) and anxiety meds to take the edge off, but believe it or not my health struggles were not over. What seemed like *totally out of left field*, so they say, my face, stomach, and sides started breaking out with something that looked like a cross between acne and hives. I knew it wasn't my normal acne, especially because it wasn't just on my face. But it also didn't look quite like the hives I usually got from forgetting to take my Zyrtec antihistamine. I was baffled, and really discouraged. I went from feeling like I was finally making a little headway with my health to dealing with yet *another* issue?! I swear I'm not a hypochondriac, although I was sure that's how people were viewing me.

I started getting the inclination (intuition maybe) to think that whatever it was might have been caused by food. I had never been diagnosed with food allergies before, but along with the skin breakouts, my stomach would start to feel uncomfortable.

I didn't want to make another doctor appointment. Around that same time I had seen ads for several at-home lab testing companies marketing that you could take labs and get results quickly and from the comfort of your own home. Seemed legit and convenient – more convenient than going to my primary care doctor to get a referral to going to a specialist who would probably send me to get labs done, then waiting for labs results, then going back to discuss lab results… (sigh). So I bought one, a food sensitivity test. Results – I was sensitive to 22 foods! And they were really hard to avoid foods – practically everything dairy, baker's and brewer's yeast (everything bread), coffee (that was the worst!), yogurt, garlic, some shell fish varieties, and several other random foods, everything from spices to artichokes. So I could eat leaves and meat.

Really?!?! How could this be happening to me?! After those results came back I felt like I had to make a doctor appointment. So I went from my primary care doctor to a new allergist. She explained the difference between food "allergies" and "sensitivities", or "intolerances". Both deal with jacked up immune systems, but the term *allergies* tend to be used when symptoms are much more serious (like anaphylaxis), whereas *sensitives* are milder, but both involve your body incorrectly reacting negatively to something you consume.

Once again I went into that appointment prepared with all my notes. In the end she recommended I do an "elimination diet". I remember doing a lot of, *uh huh, okay, umm hmm* and head nodding in the appointment, then crying in the parking lot as I walked to my car. Did she not hear me when I said that I work full-time and have four little kids?! She thinks I have time to do an elimination diet?! I could barely find time to brush my teeth twice a day – and flossing, forget it.

My Second Miracle – Low Dose Naltrexone (LDN)

Finding out about my second key "shift" (miracle) has been thanks to my dad. One of his brothers, my Uncle Tim, has been battling with multiple sclerosis for several years now. So my dad has done a lot of research on treatments to help him. Second miracle – Low Dose Naltrexone (LDN). This miracle drug was discovered in 1980 by Dr. Ian Zagon and was first used in higher doses to help drug addicts in their recovery. Fast forward a few years, patient trials revealed it could also benefit chronic and autoimmune diseases (PCOS, like MS and many others, is autoimmune). Autoimmune = dysfunctional immune system. "LDN is a safe, non-toxic and inexpensive drug that helps regulate a dysfunctional immune system" (ldnresearchtrust.org). First of all, no one ever told me PCOS was autoimmune. That was something else I learned on my own, thanks again to YouTube. Upon knowing it was autoimmune, my dad started wondering if LDN could help me as well. My Uncle Tim's MS had been responding well to it, so we started thinking that maybe I could give it a try.

Insert Dr. Schmeidler. She was my wonderful Catholic primary care doctor I mentioned before. I was thankful to her for being open to allowing me to experiment with LDN. By that time, as you can imagine, I had really lost faith in doctors and in our overall "health" care system in general. For people who are in great health, awesome. Our current system probably works for them. Once a year physical and access to labs and meds for whenever they're sick. For someone who's chronically ill, it usually means a dozen or so different people (doctors and nurses) who don't know or talk to each other, who work in different buildings, use different digital systems, all trying different things, each focusing on one body system (because body systems are separate and don't have anything to do with each other – insert another eye roll), sending you in different directions, and it can feel like the right hand doesn't know what the left hand is doing. Our "health" care system can be as dysfunctional as a dysfunctional immune system, actually. Not one person's fault, just the way the system (of a huge country) has become over the years, I suppose.

Why am I saying all this? Because I came to realize that no one was in control of my health but me. I had to be my #1 advocate. If something didn't work, it had to be me who recognized it, sounded the alarm, and perused other options. I will not be a victim, because victim-mentality will not get me anywhere! It's just a shame that chronically ill people sometimes go years (decades in my case) before they're properly diagnosed and prescribed the right remedies to help them.

In my case, I'm so incredibly thankful that Dr. Schmeidler was willing to take a risk with me and prescribe LDN. I say *risk*, not because LDN is dangerous – quite the contrary, it's very harmless if it doesn't work for someone – but risk in the sense that it really hasn't been used much to treat PCOS, so research is still up and coming.

Regardless, Dr. Schmeidler and I took the plunge together and I started taking between 1 and 10 mg every night before bed.

A couple things to note about my journey with LDN so far. I read (and watched on YouTube) that some people can have crazy vivid dreams during the first several weeks. That never happened to me. I did realize, though, that taking lower doses (like 1-4 mg) was better for me and made me less sleepy. You might be wondering about the varying doses. For me it actually works best when I alter the dosage slightly each evening. I do this on my own with a simple pill cutter. What I've read is that for some people, taking the exact same dose every night can somehow

allow your immune system to get too used to that dose and cause
unwanted side effects like sleepiness (immune system not
functioning optimally), which is exactly what started happening to
me after about four months of taking the same dose. Slightly
altering the dosage can result in "keeping your immune system on
its toes" and not getting too used to it. Some nights I purposefully
don't take it at all.

For most people, side effects are minimal – much more
convenient (and healthy) than many drugs that come with a list of
possible side effects as long as this book. And some that are really
dangerous. Doctors be like, *"Here, take this pill to help lower
your blood pressure, but just know that you might die of a blood
clot, kidney disease, breast cancer, or a stroke. So come back in
two weeks to see if we've got your blood pressure under control!"*
That's not the case with LDN.

It's been a year since I started taking Low Dose Naltrexone
and I feel normal (meaning I feel fantastic!). I say *normal* because
I imagine this is how generally healthy, *normal*, people feel all the
time. Their thoughts aren't consumed with their health. They can
make plans without automatically thinking about how the plans
might negatively affect them physically or emotionally, or if
they'll be able to make it through the plans, or how incredibly
difficult whatever it is might be just from a constant feeling of
blah, of not feeling 100%.

Specifically, all my problems with allergies and sinuses (yes,
even after two surgeries I was still suffering) – GONE GONE
GONE. No más. For the first time in 17 years I'm off Zyrtec. I had
attempted on multiple occasions throughout the years to go off
those pills. I knew that some of the fatigue I had experienced for a
long time was due to those pills. But every time I tried to quit
taking them, around the 36 hour mark, the hives would come back,
and they were just as miserable as the first time I broke out.

No more nasal sprays. No more food sensitivities. No more
need for an air purifier. I can go for a walk outside without

breaking out in hives. I'm sleeping A LOT better. I actually have somewhat of a cycle. It's still not completely regular – the last several months they've been between the 30-40 day range (still, so much better than 70+ days). Skin looks great. I've noticed that small cuts, bruises, and scabs heal faster than they used to. I have more energy. No more brain fog. And best of all, I can actually focus more on things and people besides myself, like writing this book for instance to share my story.

It's amazing to think that such a tiny sliver of a pill before bed has had such a positive impact on my health and life. When I get to Heaven someday I'm going to hug Dr. Zagon for sharing his discovery of LDN with the world.

I swear that every week I see new YouTube videos from doctors and patients talking about the use of LDN for more and more diseases of all types. I have even seen some videos talking about its use now for weight loss and general health and longevity due to its anti-inflammatory and immune-boosting powers.

In the most basic terms, LDN works by stimulating the body to produce more endorphins, and healthy levels of endorphins = happy and healthy body and mind and stronger immune system. And stronger immune system = less inflammation. Makes me wonder how much of our population could use just a little LDN in their life. Especially given the pandemic and our high-stress lifestyles, *who doesn't need a little boost in their endorphin levels now a days??* By the way, low endorphin levels are very much attributed to the brain inflammation I mentioned earlier.

I don't mean to downgrade the immense complexities involved with our anatomy and physiology, nor the research or researchers who have spent years, decades, and even lifetimes studying the human body. I am not a doctor or scientist. I am someone who has been plagued by a chronic illness and has learned through trial, error, self-advocacy, research, determination, and prayer how to overcome it.

I will end this chapter with this thought – *I wonder what percentage of doctors are trying LDN with their patients in comparison to other medicines that have more dangerous side effects? How many patients just need a stronger immune system to get to the root cause of their health issues?*

Chapter 4

OTHER LIFESTYLE CHOICES THAT HELP ME KEEP THE DISEASE IN CHECK

Besides my two miracles – the Creighton Model and LDN – there are numerous other tricks, strategies, and *ah ha's* I've come to realize throughout my struggles and journey with PCOS. I'm still learning, but after lots of research and experimentation, I have found a few of these lifestyle tweaks to be absolute non-negotiables for me to keep the disease in check, especially <u>intermittent fasting, heat therapy, vitamin D, limiting sugar, taking the right supplements, and exercise</u>. I'm certain the others help as well to a smaller degree, but those help me the most. And I do believe that PCOS cannot be cured or managed without a focus on improved lifestyle.

Please don't let yourself feel overwhelmed when reading through my list of lifestyle tweaks. If a few tricks that have helped me sound like something you could try to incorporate into your life, great! Don't feel like you have to do a complete 180 and try them all at once. Slow and steady wins the race. And remember to give yourself several months to start noticing differences – at least three.

The last pages of the book offer a simple planning framework organized by these considerations, if that could be helpful to you in getting started.

Intermittent Fasting

#1 for me hands down is intermittent fasting. If you haven't researched the benefits of fasting, you definitely should. I follow two amazing doctors on YouTube – Dr. Mindy Pelz and Dr. Sten Ekberg who talk about this topic and the countless benefits it offers – everything from fat burning and weight loss, to hormone regulation, even curing cancer and chronic diseases! No joke – watch their videos and give intermittent fasting a try – I promise you won't regret it. Two things it really helps to lower – insulin and inflammation, and PCOS sufferers need to be extra mindful of their insulin and inflammation levels. *Every woman with PCOS has insulin resistance!*

You will learn there are many different ways to fast. For me, I prefer a daily 16:8 ratio – I fast for 16 hours and only eat within an 8 hour window. The schedule that works best for me is not eating after 8:00 pm and not before noon the next day. But I don't drive myself crazy with this. If I have evening plans, for instance, I might eat after 8:00 pm. The next day I might try to extend the fast beyond noon, or sometimes I don't. No big deal, I'll just pick back up the next day, or as soon as I can. Some people prefer longer fasting periods less frequently (autophagy), such as 24-48 hour fasts (or more) once a week, as an example.

There are some select foods and beverages that will not break a fast if consumed, like black coffee and herbal tea. That for sure helps me in the morning when I feel like I just need a little something to sip on. And honestly, after a day or two of starting this new routine, your hunger pains will go away. Sometimes if I'm feeling extra out-of-whack, I'll fast for a longer period of time (autophagy) to give my body extra time to heal (aka lower inflammation).

It's actually good to be hungry, believe it or not. People really don't need to (and shouldn't) eat nearly as frequently as we are accustomed to nowadays in the U.S. Meal, snack, sugary drink, meal, snack, sugary drink, meal, snack, sugary drink – *constantly.* Despite what many prominent (*cough cough – national*) health organizations tell you, breakfast is not the most important meal of the day and eating more frequently will not help your metabolism in any way shape or form. There has never been any research to support those claims, despite what we've been told for decades now via commercials, ads, and deceptive food labels by greedy food manufacturing companies.

Fasting can help in so many ways with your health, but it does require discipline to change your habits. When making any lifestyle change, we can't ignore our psychology (mind – body – spirit – they are intertwined, not separate). So if you struggle with discipline in other areas of your life, you will need to focus on improving that first, otherwise failure is inevitable. Seriously, subscribe to those YouTube doctors and start watching their videos.

Heat Therapy

This remedy is also connected to insulin resistance. And, again, EVERY woman with PCOS is insulin resistant. Insulin resistance = too much glucose (sugar) in your blood. Too much glucose in your blood does damage to the walls of your veins and arteries. That damage leads to poor blood flow (circulation). Poor blood flow directly and indirectly leads to high blood pressure, triglycerides, cholesterol, and low oxygen levels in the blood.

Insert heat therapy. Imagine frozen water inside a hose. As the water is heated, it runs faster and smoother. That is what heat therapy does to our veins and arteries. It improves blood flow and oxygen. Healthy circulation and blood oxygen levels are essential for good egg health and ovulation. And remember from the previous chapters…curing PCOS is all about making sure we ovulate!

There are many ways to use heat therapy. I bought an electric heating pad off Amazon. Every night I turn it on the highest level and lay it over my lower abdomen for about fifteen minutes while I read or watch tv. I swear that I noticed my waist circumference get smaller after just a few weeks of doing this every night. And I am 100% sure it is helping my ovary and egg health, making it more likely that I will ovulate every month, <u>which, again, is the goal!</u>

Coffee can be very bad for me if I'm not careful with how I drink it, which really stinks because I love coffee. Too much of it wreaks havoc on my body – makes my insulin levels go up, makes me anxious, and dries out my skin. I have no doubt that our Starbucks lifestyle today plays a *huge* role in women's health issues. For one, coffee can make a women's androgen levels higher than they should be. Again, remember the title, ***Xeno— Estro—Andro—Testo—WHAT?!*** Androgens are male hormones. All women have a small amount of androgens, just like all men have a small amount of estrogen. But when a women's androgen levels get too high, it's not good. And coffee can unfortunately be a culprit for some women, *especially if it contains loads of sugar and creamer!*

A couple alterations I do to allow me to still enjoy it while also listening to my body – buy tiny coffee mugs, like the 1950's size mugs. Every year our dishes get bigger and bigger while our bodies are screaming *smaller please*! Besides that, drink it black or with a tiny bit of natural sugar – no fake sugar (sucralose is one of many ultra-processed inflammation-inducing sugars and it gives me headaches btw, and be careful because they sneak it into a lot of "healthy" drinks). One tiny cup of joe a day only during my follicular phase (after period, before ovulation) when I'm trying to get my body to ovulate (remember, ovulation = progesterone production = *yay*). I sometimes replace coffee with lemon balm or spearmint tea during those days, which are next on my list.

Lemon Balm & Spearmint

Lemon Balm is an herb in the mint family that I consume regularly for its antianxiety, anti-stress, and sleep-inducing benefits. It is anti-inflammatory, antibacterial, antiviral, and is a go-to herb in many cultures of the world as a result. Studies have shown that on average, people feel the calming benefits of lemon balm within one to three hours of consuming it as a tea or supplement, or applying it as an essential oil to the skin (I prefer the tea).

Another herb in the mint family is spearmint. In Spanish spearmint is called *yerba buena* – the "good herb", and there's a reason for that. Spearmint is so good for women needing to balance their hormones! Remember the thing about androgen levels being too high? Spearmint magically fixes that. And it's also really high in antioxidants that help lower oxidative stress. Several studies have been conducted with results proving that spearmint is great for women with PCOS because it decreases testosterone and, in turn, increases LH (luteinizing hormone), FSH (follicle-stimulating hormone), and estradiol.

How do I know when my androgen levels are too high? Remember the black hairs? Yep – my unwanted black hairs start to come back. So as soon as I start to see them on my upper lip, chin, right breast, and stomach, I know I need to up my spearmint intake. Bonus – you may not have to shave as often either because your other bodily hairs might also decrease.

There are several ways to take spearmint – drink it as a tea, soak in Epsom salts with added spearmint (or you can just throw a few spearmint tea bags in your bath water), or rub spearmint oil on your skin. Topical (skin) absorption can actually yield more benefits versus ingesting a tea, which has to pass through your digestive system. It does take a few months to see a significant difference. In fact, it may take up to three menstrual cycles before a woman notices significant differences from any treatment or lifestyle change she makes to balance hormones.

Back to spearmint. I buy tea and Epsom salts on Amazon and I also grow my own. It's so easy to grow, inside or outside. If you grow your own, place about five large leaves with the stem in boiling water and steep for about five minutes. I drink mine plain, but if you need a little extra sweetness, add a bit of locally grown organic honey. Locally grown is best because the bees in your area pollinate local plants, which gives you exposure to those plants and can lessen your chances of plant allergies.

Vitamin D

Another way for women to naturally lower androgen levels and balance hormones is by making sure they have enough of the sunshine vitamin – vitamin D. Growing research suggests that women with metabolic disturbances and insulin resistance (which, again, may be the culprit of PCOS) have a vitamin D deficiency. What I have noticed over the years is that my cycles are much better (less PMS and more regular) in the late spring and summer. I believe that has everything to do with the amount of natural vitamin D from the sun I get during those months. So much so that I do not need to supplement during that time. But come late summer when the kiddos are back in school and I am no longer at the pool or outside nearly as much, my vitamin D levels start to decrease. That's when I start supplementing. Who knows, maybe there are other substances from the sun that our bodies need and that science hasn't discovered yet.

Something else I do during the fall and winter – I lay down on the floor where the sun is shining through a window to soak up some vitamin D – rich rays without having to go outside in the freezing cold. It feels so good doing that, and I can feel my body (and my mind) thanking me. Naturally, the more skin I have exposed, the more D I have soaking into my system. We have to remember that we are not creatures of the deep blue sea or cave dwelling bats – our bodies require the sun. Considering the amount of time many people spend inside now a days, it's no surprise that more and more people (men and women) are deficient in vitamin D. I do apply a mineral-based sun screen to be sure I'm protecting myself from the dangerous UV rays.

Sugar is Poison!

Before I start on sugar, just know that sometimes I have weaknesses in this area! How many decades now have we been saying that processed sugar is poison? But really. Sugar is <u>so</u> <u>so</u> <u>so</u> bad. For everyone. It wreaks HAVOC on the microbiomes in our tummies. And we've known for quite a while that our gut microbiome is kind of important. Hippocrates himself said 2,500 years ago that all disease starts in our gut!

Sadly, we Americans put sugar in literally everything, not just candy and desserts. Milk, ketchup, bacon. Whose brilliant idea was it to dip hot greasy bacon in chocolate?! Americans are so addicted to sugar. I would venture to say there are more Americans addicted to sugar than drugs and alcohol. And believe it or not, sugar has the same effect on our brains as consuming drugs and alcohol does. Many of my friends and family from other countries have commented on how much sweeter everything tastes in the United States. *Why?* Because we add tons of sugar to *everything*! As if Twinkies don't have enough poison (added sugar and preservatives) on their own – now we have to deep fry them and cover them in chocolate?!

Because PCOS sufferers, like sufferers of other autoimmune and chronic illnesses, have a higher tendency to leaky gut and inflammation, sugar intake really needs to be kept at a minimum. And if you're someone like me who gets sugar cravings, that can be really hard. But actually sugar cravings are a sign of unbalanced hormones.

One really helpful thing I do if I've eaten too much sugar (besides intermittent fasting) – drink the syrup made from combining white or red onion and sugar. I know what you're thinking – *What?! To help lower blood sugar you want me to drink sugar? With onions?* The answer is yes. It isn't a hocus pocus witch's potion – it's a legit natural way to lower blood sugar levels (and it also helps with colds and coughs). YouTube it.

I don't want to be a hypocrite, though. Full disclosure – "eat less sugar" is in the category of "do as I say not as I do" – I still need to get better at this. It's so hard to not eat sugar! But I'm trying. I definitely have less PMS when I have less sugar in my body.

By the way, I'm not talking about healthy, natural sugars like the ones we get from cinnamon, honey, fruits, and other <u>plants</u>. Yes, our bodies need sugar to fuel multiple body systems. Without it, we die. I'm talking about refined, processed, "added" sugars. Companies unnecessarily add them to their products so they taste better and so you're more likely to buy them again – simple. (I can hear my four little munchkins in my head begging for more Lucky Charms as I'm writing this.). Our generation and our kids' generations have been conditioned since childhood to be addicted to sugar. If you're not in the habit of checking food labels for "added sugars", you should be. It tells you just that – how much sugar has been added to the product (beyond the natural sugar amount). Then google a picture to get a visual of how much sugar that is. If 30 grams of sugar in your cup of yogurt didn't already seem outrageous, it will once you get a visual.

I try to only buy products that have little-to-no added sugars. Yes, they do exist. Are they hard to find? Kind of. But companies are making more and more healthy options as time goes on. I like shopping at *Fresh Thyme* and *Aldi's*. They have plenty of desert options with very little added sugars. You can even find low sugar options at cheaper places like *Dollar General* – you just have to spend a few minutes reading labels.

Berries

Another suggestion if you get sugar cravings is berries with honey and plain yogurt. The antioxidants in berries are so good for everyone. The reason why I eat as many berries as possible is because they are great at reducing oxidative stress, which is basically prolonged elevated cortisol levels. Remember all my comments about cortisol? I have come to learn that my self-criticizing, idealistic, people-pleasing perfectionist self probably has somewhat of a natural tendency to high cortisol levels (aka I stress myself out easily). It's part of who I am. I want to make the world a better place. I want to be the very best I can be at everything. Sounds great, right? Not exactly. It's so stressful being that way!!! If you're a perfectionist, you know exactly what I'm talking about. If you're not, I'm happy for you. I don't wish it on anyone. In a way, having kids has helped me lighten up. Somedays the dishes just aren't going to be done before everyone goes to bed. And who cares, really? We have a bed to sleep on and we're going to bed happy. The dishes can wait til tomorrow. But despite my efforts to chill more often, I still have a ways to go.

Back to berries. Three tips if you want to increase your berry consumption to help you decrease oxidative stress. Buy the frozen bags, you get more bang for your buck. If you are someone who spends $5 at Target on a tiny bag of dried strawberries, buy an air fryer or a food dehydrator and make them yourself. You can even use the frozen ones to do this, just let them thaw first. And finally, grow your own! In my growing zone (zone 6), they are perennials. I've recently started growing blueberries and raspberries and have already harvested some! I'm feeling somewhat like a modern day Hunter Gatherer – walking out to my backyard, picking and eating wild (homegrown) berries. They are low maintenance and they grow pretty fast if planted in the right spot.

Hydroponic Gardening

I'm just starting to dabble with indoor hydroponic gardening, so I can't give as much advice with this one. But I can tell you after watching tons of YouTube videos that it has a lot of potential to positively impact our health. If there's a little sarcasm to the voice inside your head wondering how gardening could ever help with PCOS, hear me out. In a nutshell, hydroponic gardening is growing crops with water, sunlight, and a few key minerals mixed into the water. That's right – no soil. People are growing their own food sources (mainly vegetables and herbs) inside the comfort of their own homes – no pesticides, no GMOs, no weather dependency, no farmer dependency – just you, your windows (or grow lights), water, and your nutrient-rich crops!

Like I said, I've just started this new journey. I have small, simple growing systems on the windowsills in my kitchen and bathroom, and I've been making mini greenhouses out of recycled plastic containers and ziplock bags. My bok choy "microgreens" are growing and sprouting seeds like crazy. Every couple days my kids help me pick the leaves for mini salads. By the way, new research shows that microgreens are incredibly nutritious, more nutrient-dense actually than their mature counterparts. For all these reasons, I'm excited and eager to continue this little experiment I've got going to better ensure a daily intake of nutrient-rich, preservative-free microgreens.

H_2O

Are you drinking enough water? Probably not. PCOS sufferers need to drink lots of it – like lots. Remember the connection between PCOS and metabolic syndrome? Drinking enough fluids is important for everyone, especially for people with chronic health conditions like metabolic syndrome and insulin resistance. And it's the easiest, cheapest change you can make. Look for a big water jug that has time markings labeled on the outside showing how much you should have gulped down by those times of the day. It's an easy way to help keep you on track. If you don't care for lugging around a giant water jug that doesn't fit in your car's cup holders, I bought one on Amazon that is 1000 ml (four cups) with a marker/reminder at the bottom to refill halfway through the day. It has a built-in fruit diffuser to add a bit of natural flavor, too

Speaking of flavor, be cautious of flavored bottled water and flavor-enhancing liquids meant to be added to plain water. While the packaging and nutrition labels may seem harmless, or even "healthy", they usually sneak in chemicals and/or ultra-processed sugars like sucralose and other artificial sweeteners that are not good at all for you. Remember my comment about sucralose giving me headaches? It can also raise insulin and blood sugar levels in some people, and it is very bad for our gut biome. If drinking plain water is not your thing, flavor it with fruit and/or mint leaves. I squeeze lemon and lime in my water and add spearmint leaves and blueberries, all of which have antioxidants. I also add chia seeds to get my omegas. One more word of caution about drinking more water – just make sure it's not heavy-metal-infested tap water you're drinking (I'm speaking from experience – more on that in #6 of the next chapter).

An added bonus to increasing your water intake – it's great for your skin. Since I've battled with acne and rosacea practically as long as I've been battling my dysfunctional hormones, I have a few additional tips to share at the end of this chapter beyond drinking more water that have been monumental in helping me get my skin issues under control.

Supplements

Remember me saying that at one point my entire cabinet was filled with vitamin and supplement bottles? I've tried them all. Hands down the best of the best is a mental wellness company called *Amare Global*. I'm pretty sure my body, especially my digestive system, might still be recovering from so many years of constant antibiotics for sinus infections and skin issues. *Amare Global* supplements have been very good for me. They only use plants that are proven to balance our gut microbiome and our "gut-brain axis". For years, mental health has largely focused on our brain. What if I were to tell you that your GUT (not your brain) produces 95% of your serotonin, just as an example? So many of our physiological processes start in our GUT (not our brain). With that in mind, and knowing how poor our diet is today, it's no wonder we're in the midst of a mental health crisis!!

They have a lot of options to choose from. I currently take their "Happy Hormones Trio", and I can tell you that my hormones are, in fact, very happy thanks to them. No more bloating, little-to-no PMS, and my energy is through the roof! My husband takes them as well (the male version). They are a little pricey, but worth it. Here's an idea…instead of a daily $5 Starbucks sugar bomb, use the money to try one of their supplements for a few months and you'll see what I mean.

Besides *Amare Global* supplements and my vitamin D during the cold months, one other that I can't live without is the nutritional yeast I spoke of earlier, especially for its B1 vitamins (thiamine) – a crucial vitamin that most Americans are deficient in. There are lots of YouTube videos on health complications due to B1 deficiency (Added bonus – it's really good for hair, skin, and nails.)

I mentioned nutritional yeast in the last chapter because it (along with my *Amare Global* supplements) helped me totally wean myself off my antidepressant, Lexapro. I also took CBD oil the first few weeks when I was having withdrawals, which is normal to experience when stopping an antidepressant. The CBD oil really helped me during those weeks.

In addition to what we eat, what we don't eat, and how often we eat (think intermittent fasting again), our current American lifestyle is so dysfunctional and anti-family, and that, I believe, is the #1 culprit to the rising amount of sick people that we are experiencing. This isn't the way God intends us to live…energy-drinking stressed-out workaholics always racing from one job or activity to the next, scarfing down meals in our vehicles, glued to screens, popping pills, depending on others (government) for food and "good" health, and then wondering why we keep losing our mind!?? If this resonates with you, no judgement whatsoever – I hear you. Life should be and *can* be much more enjoyable. These additional tips I'm about to share are subtle, easy, inexpensive, and they help me. Maybe they could help you too?

Sleep

Besides Low Dose Naltrexone and *Amare Global* supplements, both of which have been monumental for helping me sleep better, I have come to realize that I just need more hours of z's than the average person. I know some women who can function just fine on five hours of sleep. NOT ME. They say the average adult needs between seven and eight hours of restful quality sleep. I need more like ten, which makes sense the more I think about it. I'm a busy-body perfectionist. My mind is always racing. Something always needs to be done (*ha* – more like 1,000 things always need to be done) and can always be done better. It makes me wonder if all perfectionists require more sleep? It's so important for our bodies as they fight off all kinds of free radicals and stress (cortisol) we're exposed to these days. I've been seeing more and more articles and YouTube videos about sleep being "the new self-care", and it's true. Do you spend money on beauty products trying to preserve a youthful glow? Do you also stay up too late on your phone or tv? If you answered yes to both, I can assure you that you'll get a better bang for your buck by just turning off the screen and getting a few extra hours of sleep. If you're like me, you may have to put your phone in a different part of the room where it's out of reach til morning, otherwise I'm tempted like a teenager to reach for it and do a little more scrolling (aka a little less sleeping).

One more thing I do to help me sleep better – make banana tea. Bananas have nutrients that can improve sleep – potassium, magnesium, and tryptophan, an amino acid that helps with the body's production of melatonin and serotonin. The way I make banana tea is by cutting a whole banana (peel and all) in four sections. I then cut each section open a bit to allow for easier release of nutrients into the boiling water. I boil it for ten minutes.

That's it. I usually drink it at dinner, and I also give it to my kids to help them fall asleep and stay asleep. We drink it plain as it naturally has a sweet taste to it, but honey and/or cinnamon could be added to make it even sweeter. (Also remember lemon balm mentioned in #3 that helps with sleep.)

Chronobiology

Chrono—what?? Chronobiology. It's the study of our natural physiological rhythms (our internal clock: light = day and dark = night). Think back to the whole *energy-drinking pill-popping workaholics* thing and add in all the hours the younger generations spend staring at blue light screens. Our physiology is *royally* messed up these days, again due to our *lifestyles*. Think about it. Just one hundred years ago the only way people could see after the sun went down was with a candle or fire, which does no harm to our internal clocks.

So another thing to consider if you struggle with sleep is whether or not your chronobiology (internal clock) is messed up. If it is, it could very well be tied to the screens you're staring at off and on all day. If your job demands that you stare at a screen all day, thanks to recent research and technology, you can fix it easier than ever with special blue light glasses that simulate sunlight and stimulate sensory cells in our eyes called photosensitive Retinal Ganglion Cells (ipRGCs).

I wear blue light blocking screen glasses wherever and whenever I'm staring at a screen – tv, computer, or cell phone. I know they help because my eyes don't feel nearly as strained at the end of the day when I use them. They are not for vision whatsoever. They are for blocking the harmful light from screens, which we are exposed to constantly today.

LED lights don't help our internal clocks either. They may be more efficient for our budgets, but they're not more efficient for our bodies. So if you're struggling with sleep, look into what light bulbs are being used in your home and consider the screen glasses. There is a company called *Ayo* that sells glasses specific for helping someone wake up in the morning. I haven't tried these yet but I am looking forward to testing them out soon.

Exercise

PCOS sufferers need REGULAR EXERCISE!!! But not the psycho exercise you see on *Insanity* workout videos. Remember high cortisol? Exercise is the best and easiest way to lower it. But be careful, doing insanely intense workouts can actually have the opposite effect. If you're not currently working out – start. If you already do but you're feeling like you're not making much progress, it could be because you're actually overdoing it. Like most people, my workout routine is like a rollercoaster – all over the place. Some months/weeks are better than others. But the instant I feel my body (cortisol) start screaming *HELP!,* I know I need to get back on track. If you're still not convinced, consider this – it has been proven that muscle mass is actually an indicator of longevity. *Hmmm.*

So ideally I make it to the gym 2-3 times a week. I prefer to take classes. I need someone next to me telling me to *Keep holding that plank!* to push and encourage me. Sometimes if I can't make it to the gym, I do a few minutes of stretching and a two-minute plank at home. A two-minute workout sounds pathetic, right? Wrong!! Try a two-minute plank and you'll see what I mean. It works your sides, abs, glutes, arms, back, and legs – all at the same time. If you don't have hardly any time for workouts, gradually work your way up to doing multi-minute full planks. You can start easy with your knees on the floor if needed – you will still get a good workout that way. And don't forget deep breathing!

Side note about exercise – I mentioned before that I used to be a yoga, pilates, and cycling instructor for 24 Hour Fitness gyms. While doing those workouts didn't magically cure my

PCOS, I felt pretty amazing afterwards, especially the meditation and breathing part at the end of the classes. If you haven't tried yoga or meditation before, I highly recommend you do!

As long as I keep up my fairly easy workout routine, I'm fine. But like I said, after a couple weeks go by of me "off the exercise train", I start to feel more anxious. Speaking of anxious…

Magnesium

Believe it or not, recent research (very recent – like just within the last couple years) suggests a link between PCOS and metabolic syndrome. Why is this important? Because people with metabolic syndrome often times have a magnesium deficiency. A recent theory of why this happens is insulin. Remember the *sugar is poison* thing? Chronically high insulin levels lower magnesium. With our poor diet, many people have a magnesium deficiency these days and don't even know it. And besides affecting insulin levels, other unwanted symptoms can occur, ranging from anxiety, insomnia, even more serious issues like heart palpitations. So if you're like most Americans not eating an ideal diet, you might consider a magnesium supplement.

I actually prefer a magnesium spray over pills because a spray gets absorbed by the skin very quickly, whereas a pill has to go through your digestive system and, in turn, losses its potency. A bath with Epsom salts is also another option. Whenever I feel my hormones are out of whack and my insulin might be too high (hand swelling is a key indicator for me), I reach for my magnesium spray. It can be sprayed anywhere on the skin. I prefer to spray my chest. The company I prefer is called *Ease*. I feel the benefits of their magnesium spray within minutes.

Full Body Massages

I am lucky to have an amazing massage therapist whose magic hands and talents relieve so much stress (cortisol) from my body just within an hour's time. I wish I could have it done every day. Since I can't, I actually have a device bought from a company called Ashley Black that allows me to massage my fascia in the shower, which helps relieve stress and muscle aches and pains. Fascia is the connective tissue that surrounds and holds all of our organs, nerve fibers, muscles, bones, and blood vessels in place. It's basically the glue that holds our bodies together. Within the scientific world, fascia has largely been unnoticed and understudied. Very recently it has been added as a body system – the fascia system. There are studies revealing that some people's aches and pains are more due to unhealthy fascia and less due to unhealthy or stiff muscles.

I use my fascia massager pretty regularly in the shower with cheap coconut oil so it doesn't pull on my skin. (Bonus – it is the most effective way to eliminate cellulite, because cellulite is actually unhealthy fascia.) My whole body feels better after using it. When I'm feeling extra sore and tight, that's when I call my massage therapist. The pressure points she hits relieve so much stress (cortisol). I know I sound like a broken record, but keep on remembering – chronic high stress due to lifestyle = chronic high cortisol, and chronic high cortisol = all kinds of health ailments.

Garlic

Last but definitely not least – garlic. This seemingly magic plant has a plethora of health benefits that have been well documented throughout history. It is perhaps the best plant to use regularly to strengthen our immune systems. Numerous studies have proven that regular intake of garlic significantly decreases our chances of developing the common cold, high blood pressure, heart disease, dementia and Alzheimer's, and its powerful antioxidants help to improve bone health, menopausal symptoms, detoxify the body of heavy metals, and on and so forth. So take just a few minutes to read studies involving garlic.

Besides using it for cooking, I use it medicinally in several different ways. I always have a jar filled with fermented garlic cloves and honey in the kitchen. I smash the cloves before adding them to the jar as that action releases its sulfur compounds, which is where its magic powers come from. Then I let it ferment in the honey for several days. The honey will begin to bubble as the garlic ferments. I open the lid once a day, give or take, to release the gases built up in the jar. The liquid that results is a powerful anti-bacterial, anti-viral, immune-boosting potion that my kids, husband, and I drink – one spoonful every day.

I also always have on hand a jar of garlic oil. The minute one of us begins to show signs of sickness, I put a drop in each ear and use a Q-tip to coat the inside of the nostrils with the oil. Just like magic, the symptoms subside! Take a few minutes to search for garlic oils on Amazon and read the comments. You'll be amazed at how many people have very recently discovered the healing powers of this underestimated plant (actually a vegetable, although most believe it to be an herb).

Like I said at the beginning of this chapter – don't allow yourself to feel overwhelmed! Don't allow yourself to think, "I have to go out and buy all this stuff, spend lots of money, wake up tomorrow and try living a totally different lifestyle with different habits. You will fail. Be disciplined and gradually make small changes over the course of a year or two. All of these remedies have gradually become part of my new lifestyle overtime. Remember, slow and steady always wins the race, always. If you want more step-by-step guidance with pictures of these lifestyle alterations I have made, check out my workbook, *Kick PCOS to the Curb: The PCOS Lifestyle Workbook*.

Because my PCOS has included all sorts of miserable, hormonal skin problems dating back to middle school and puberty, I have also documented five skin remedies that have 100%

changed my skin recently (and my confidence). If you or someone you know is struggling with hormonal skin issues, consider the remedies in the next chapter.

Chapter 5

MY FIVE HORMONAL PCOS SKIN SAVIORS

Tretinoin Microsphere Gel 0.04%

If I were to tell you to make one change to your facial skin routine it would be to incorporate the use of Tretinoin Microsphere Gel. You don't need to have hormonal skin problems for it to be beneficial to you. This gel helps with basically any and all skin issues from hyperpigmentation, enlarged pores, scaring, wrinkles, acne, and on and so forth. *Why and how?* It speeds up cell turnover. And as we age, our cell reproduction slows significantly.

I use the 0.04% because my skin is so sensitive, but there are stronger levels. I use it twice a week *after* applying my moisturizer at night (lessens irritation while still doing the job). And I don't apply it if I know that I'm going to be out in the sun the next day. My skin has never looked better, in large part because of this magic gel. I'm nearing 40 and my skin looks better now than it did when I was in my twenties. I buy mine from Okdermo Beauty, Health, & Skincare. It's $32 and lasts me over a year. Can't beat that.

Only Organic

It's so hard to find beauty products that have zero unnecessary ingredients. Most of those ingredients are fillers and preservatives. The only reason they're used in products is so the company can make more money. Fillers allow companies to use less of the good (more expensive) stuff and preservatives extent the product's shelf life. They don't benefit anyone's skin, and they wreak extra havoc on sensitive skin (and on our hormones). I now only use plant-based products on my skin. My all-time favorite company is *Luminance*. Their products are 100% organic, vegan, and their customer service is second to none.

B Vitamins

Two other things I know now that I wish I had known years ago when it comes to my sensitive skin – my rosacea was due in part to leaky gut (bad diet – lots of sugar – and too many antibiotics) and extremely dry skin. It didn't look dry, it was just constantly red, and no one associated the redness with dryness because it didn't flake or crack. In addition to consuming B vitamins in my supplements and daily nutritional yeast, I apply Cicaplast Balm B5 at night before bed (just during the driest months of the year) . It leaves my skin feeling so hydrated. I buy *La Roche Posay's* B5 balm.

Silk Pillowcase

Silk is way better for your skin than cotton. For one, bacteria can't thrive on silk, whereas they can on cotton. Plus, silk doesn't cause as many wrinkles as cotton. If you're a side sleeper like me, you know what it's like waking up with trenches on your face. That doesn't happen with silk. I absolutely love my silk pillowcase and will never go back to cotton.

Balancing My pH

This trick is kind of a chemistry lesson – The first thing I do when, despite my efforts, I feel a breakout coming on (which hardly ever happens now thanks to getting my gut and hormones balanced!) is rebalance my skin's pH. What's the magic (cheap) potion to doing that – green tea mixed with a little apple cider vinegar! Another possible reason for breakouts besides bacteria overgrowth, dehydration, clogged pores, and leaky gut (sheesh, our skin can be so tricky) could be that your pH is out of whack. Our skin naturally has a pH around 4.5 – 5.5, which is slightly acidic. So the reason why green tea and apple cider vinegar mixed together works wonders is not rocket science – the pH of those two combined ingredients is about the same as our skin's pH. Apple cider vinegar is mildly acidic and green tea is mildly alkaline, so combining the two results in a perfect 4.5 – 5.5 Ph. I get both my ACV and green tea (straight green tea – no added flavors or ingredients) from Dollar General (that surely doesn't break the bank!). You can soak a washcloth in the cooled liquid and just place it over your face for a few minutes. Or, you can actually buy a bag full of eco-friendly plain masks, which is what I prefer. I steep the tea, add about a teaspoon of ACV, toss in the mask, and let it cool for a few hours. After I wash my face before bed, I put the mask on for just a few minutes, usually while I'm brushing kids' teeth and getting them ready for bed.

Rose water toner also works wonders for balancing my pH. The skin care company mentioned in #2, *Luminance*, has a great rose water toner. The second I spray it on my face much of my redness goes away. I love it so much that I could easily go through a full bottle every couple days, which is why I also use the green tea and ACV mask (more affordable). I also have a rose bush in my front yard and sometimes make a homemade rose water toner with aloe vera juice from my aloe plant and filtered water. Speaking of filtered water…

I have realized recently how acidic the tap water is in my house, which is why it's so important for me to use a pH balancing toner after washing my face. If you're wondering what the pH level is of the water in your house, you can buy test strips for about $5 on Amazon. They can be used to test tap water and also to test skin care products (face and body). I did that and threw out all products that were too acidic or too alkaline, which were causing my skin to be irritated. Typically products that are too acidic = oil and acne, and products that are too alkaline = dryness (cracking and flaking). I discovered the importance of paying attention to the pH level of water and products I put on my face just very recently, and I believe that learning about this has had a positive impact on my skin's health.

My water is so contaminated with heavy metals that my husband and I purchased a filter system for our kitchen and showerhead. The showerhead we purchased is from Crystal Quest. I researched and found theirs to be the most effective, efficient, and affordable. The first time I took a shower after installing their filter (which was a breeze), I noticed such a difference in my skin and hair. I didn't even need to apply lotion to my skin afterwards because it didn't feel dry like it normally did after showering.

I sincerely hope that some of these tricks I've learned over time can help you too. I'm thankful to have had access to information and research that have allowed me to be my own advocate – and be an advocate for my daughters as well, as they will be reaching puberty in just a few years. I hope and pray that what I know now about my own body and lifestyle will help me navigate decisions for their health and well-being. Allow me to share somethings I do with my girls (and a few that I do with my son as well) in hopes to avoid, if possible, them developing PCOS or other reproductive diseases in the future.

Chapter 6

RAISING THREE DAUGHTERS WHO MAY ALSO BE PREDISPOSED TO ACQUIRING THE DISEASE

ARE THERE WAYS TO AVOID IT??

For my husband and me, parenting means getting our four kids to heaven and teaching them the joy of helping others during our short time on this earth. I know, that's pretty heavy. But as long as we remember these long-term goals, everything else always falls into place. We don't care if our kids turn into professional athletes, CEO's, or doctors. We don't care how much money they will make in their careers. We care about them loving and serving God, knowing how to overcome adversities, survive on their own and be independent, and how to find joy in everything they do.

Of course we treat our son and our three daughters very differently. For our son, we are always instilling in him the responsibility of taking good care of his sisters, even though one of his sisters is older than him – it is his responsibility as "the boy" to protect and stand up for them. That responsibility empowers him and makes him feel special and needed. But this chapter is more about specific parenting tactics I use with my three "estrogen littles" to hopefully avoid, if possible, them having the same struggles I had growing up.

Each new generation has increased access to knowledge, thanks in large part to the internet. Long gone are the days when common folk had to rely on educated people to find answers to their problems. No – I'm not advocating against seeing specialists; I'm simply reiterating that everyone has 24/7 access to loads of information, literally at their fingertips on their cell phones. With this in mind, parents have the responsibility to reflect on their own childhood, what worked and didn't work so well, and what new information and research is available to help us make informed decisions as they relate to our kids' development.

By the way, I'm far from deserving of the mother-of-the-year award. It's easy to say and write these things – a lot harder to actually *do* them. Some days I do them better than others. But I'm trying. And each day is a new beginning. God knows I am trying and that I have good intentions.

My tips and ideas for parents to consider are grouped into three different categories – mind, body, and spirit. If one of these parts of us suffers, our whole body suffers. So we need to be sure we are nurturing all three of them in our mini-me's.

Healthy Mind (Less Stress – Cortisol)

Two words to describe everything in this category – *no stress (cortisol)*. Of course we need to teach our girls how to cope and how to overcome adversities, but too many kids are growing up today with chronic stress. Living with chronic stress and learning to overcome adversity are two very different things. Let kids be kids. Each year it seems their backpacks get heavier, evenings and weekends get busier, there's less time for playing outside, even snow days have been taken away from some kids since e-Learning as become a thing thanks to the Covid pandemic. For God sakes, let them have snow days! But unless you're a school superintendent, I'm not preaching to you about snow days. Here's what I mean exactly when I say *no stress* – and a few things I try to keep in mind as best I can as I parent my three girls (and actually these tips are also good for boys).

Don't overly control them

Doing so will likely turn them into FARTS – fanatic, anxious, rebellious teens. Trust me, you don't want to have a house full of farts in a few years. Let them make choices when appropriate. Let them make mistakes. It might not be appropriate to allow them to choose where to go on vacation, for instance (until they get older), but allow them some say in the planning. They will likely appreciate the responsibility, especially if you start when they are young. The more we allow them to feel in control of their lives from an early age, the more empowered they will feel as they get older. If the opposite happens and they feel too controlled, not only will they turn into FARTS – they will likely not feel empowered or confident, and kids with low confidence can manifest into all sorts of negative behaviors that can unfortunately last a lifetime.

Key questions you might ask yourself to see how you're faring in the control category – Are you a control freak in certain areas of your life? If yes, could parenting be one of them? Have you allowed your kids to make any decisions today? Or do you just tell them what to do all the time? There are usually psychological reasons behind an overly controlling individual – sometimes they themselves were overly controlled growing up, or maybe they experienced some sort of trauma, which can also make us want to control things too heavily. In parenting, there is a very delicate balance between freedom and control that should always be changing, depending on the kids' age. Just be mindful that the pendulum isn't leaning too far one way – giving them too much freedom or being too controlling. No one, absolutely no one likes to be controlled, and that feeling of being controlled can definitely lead to unwanted and unnecessary stress (cortisol).

No mirrors

Mirror, mirror on the wall, thanks for pointing out all of my imperfections. For some girls, mirrors are not a big deal. But be very careful, parents – especially if your girls have a tendency towards perfectionism and/or vanity. Two of my three daughters are very care free when it comes to physical appearance. They glance in the mirror for two seconds after having their hair brushed and say it looks great (aka *I don't care, just let me go play!*). The other one, though (the oldest), is already showing signs of being a perfectionist like her mommy.

I remember having a childhood vanity in my room, like many girls. It's a staple piece of feminine furniture in many homes. As I said earlier, for some girls mirrors are just mirrors. For me, and seemingly now for my oldest, three large mirrors in my room equaled three angles of seeing every possible bodily imperfection – and fixating on them until they were "perfect" in my mind. That vanity was not healthy for me. It just caused me to be more self-conscious. And remember, self-consciousness = more stress (cortisol). Any little hair that was out of place had to be fixed. And don't get me started on my acne. My vanity mirrors weren't the magnifying type, but they might as well have been in my pubescent hormonal mind. Every pimple was as large as my whole face according to the way I saw them.

So what am I getting at here? Maybe reflect on your house. It seems houses now a days come with more mirrors than cabinets and drawers. Shouldn't be a surprise, I guess. We Americans are all about me, myself and I. Do you have too many mirrors in your house? Do you see that affecting your daughters (or sons)? Seeing how our oldest is with mirrors, my husband and I have already talked about replacing the huge bathroom mirrors with smaller ones. And no mirrors in bedrooms. What purpose do they serve, especially if there are mirrors in the bathrooms?

Mirror, mirror on the wall, God loves me just the way I am, and that's all that matters.

Lavender essential oils

Lavender, along with other essential oils, has a very calming effect on our minds. I spray it in my kids' bedrooms every night before they go to sleep and I really believe it helps them fall asleep and stay asleep. I used to have an oil diffuser in their room but little hands kept spilling it, so I switched to an organic spray. Sometimes if I am sensing that one of them is overly stressed or anxious, I'll open up one of my essential oils and give it to them to just sniff on for a minute or two. Our sense of smell can be very powerful, and sometimes neglected in comparison to our other senses.

Healthy Body (More Plants)

By now I'm sure you've gotten a sense of how important diet, exercise, sleep, and relaxation are for keeping PCOS (umm…and most diseases) at bay. I don't want to wait until my girls hit puberty to feed their bodies what they need most. I am constantly reiterating to them the importance of eating healthy and taking care of their bodies. I don't stress them out when teaching them these things. I just subtly ask them to remind me what it means to eat healthy (and unhealthy).

Daily greens

My husband and I really try hard to make sure our kids eat greens every day. For us, the easiest way to do this is by putting them in soups/stews, quesadillas, and smoothies. Our main green staples are avocados, spinach, cilantro, parsley, zucchini, lime, green peppers, our bok choy microgreens, and a variety of chiles. We have never catered to our kids' desires when it comes to food – you eat what you are given or you don't eat. I believe that instilling that mindset in them from an early age has been key in helping us form them into non-picky eaters.

I'm sorry parents, but most kids are picky eaters because their parents unknowingly and inadvertently shape them into being that way. If this is speaking to you and you want to make an effort at getting your kids to eat healthier so they grow healthier (and are less likely to develop diseases), it will be difficult at first, but keep at it. Make small changes and be consistent. Empower them to love growing plants themselves. There are sadly millions of kids who go to bed hungry every night and do not die in their sleep. If your kids don't like eating healthy, they don't have to eat. Give them a few hours with an empty stomach and they'll miraculously be dying to eat veggies all of the sudden lol!

Limit sugar and fried foods

There's not a lot more to say here, as I've already covered it in previous chapters, and we've been saying it for decades now. Sugar and fried foods are poison (unless the fried foods are fried with healthy oils like avocado, olive, or coconut oil – then that's ok). Most foods are fried with ultra-refined hydrogenated oils, which are very bad for us. There are tons of yummy recipes we have access to online now a days that use healthy ingredients. No excuses here – limit giving your kids sugar and fried foods and they will thank you for it someday. You will thank yourself, too, when you have less doctor visits, fewer medical bills, and more $ in the bank.

Limit antibiotics

Because I believe that my body is in some way still suffering from having been given waaaaay too many antibiotics over the years, I'm very, very careful not to give them to my kids unless it's totally necessary. The more our bodies can recover from illnesses on their own, the stronger our immune systems become over time. Using antibiotics messes with our gut bacteria (gives us leaky gut) and suppresses our immune system – double whammy.

Plant-based medicine when possible

I use plant-based medicine as much as possible. I'm not opposed to western (synthetic) medicine at times, but I believe wholeheartedly in plants being our medicine whenever possible. When our kids get sick with a virus, I give them garlic (fermented in honey – one spoonful a day), lemon, mullein, and oregano – all of which have anti-viral properties. For tummy troubles we reach for the chamomile tea, spearmint, peppermint, and lime (all of which we grow ourselves). For allergies, skin issues, and cold/flu-like symptoms, we use echinacea, calendula, mullein, and garlic. We also regularly have a mason jar of onion and sugar syrup available to help with blood sugar levels, coughs, and sniffles. A spoonful of onion syrup = less cough and snot – winner winner chicken dinner.

One more natural remedy we use often is Epsom salts. We are careful not to put too much in their bathwater since their bodies are little, but the added minerals soaked up through their skin give them extra strength to fight off whatever ailments they are experiencing, especially during the cold months when they are outside less.

I like to think these remedies help. Of course they get sick from time to time, but overall our kids are healthy and energetic and they seem to recuperate very quickly, so I do believe they work.

Healthy Spirit (More Jesus)

Finally, if their little spirits aren't also being nourished, believe it or not, that can have a negative impact on their minds and bodies as well. As we are Catholic, we constantly pray with our kids throughout the day, every day. In the morning we say thank you Jesus for this new day. We thank Him before meals, we ask for protection whenever and wherever we drive (Our Lady of the Highway prayer), and before bedtime we pray the Hail Mary, Guardian Angel prayer, and Act of Contrition to ask for pardon for our sins we committed during the day.

If this sounds overwhelming, I promise you it is the exact opposite. Our kids at their young ages already feel a close relationship to God (Diosito), Jesus (Jesusín), Mary (Nuestra Madre Morenita), and their Guardian Angel (Ángel de la Guarda). It is comforting knowing that despite who is with them physically, they *always, always* have the Devine to turn to for help, and this frees them from anxiety, stress (cortisol), fear, and gives them peace of mind.

It also really helps to instill the joy of helping others from a young age as we are always praying for others – our families, the sick, the poor, the lonely, and everyone who is unhappy or worried about something. Anytime we pass an ambulance or police car when we are driving, they always shout out, *We need to pray for the people who need help and for the people who are helping them! (¡Tenemos que rezar por ellos!)* I love hearing them shout that out with such passion and enthusiasm, like it is partially our responsibility to help them (because as Catholics we believe that it is our responsibility to help those in need – Catholic Social Teachings). My husband and I realize that our greatest accomplishment on earth may not be something we do ourselves, but someone we raise.

Despite the struggle of sometimes getting them to behave, we also bring them to Mass with us on Sunday evenings. While it is a struggle – sometimes seemingly the hardest hour of our week – my husband and I know that our sacrifice will pay off when they are older. Receiving the sacraments, especially the Eucharist, is the #1 gift Jesus gave us that protects us from evil. If you believe in the Bible and in the four Gospels, which are accounts documented by the apostles of Jesus' life, He said to His followers, "Truly, truly I say to you, unless you eat the flesh of the Son of man and drink His blood, you have no life in you. John 6:53".

Why would parents go to great lengths to protect their children physically and mentally but not spiritually? Or pray with them but purposefully withhold the Eucharist from them (their greatest protection)? Our bodies and minds will be gone before we know it, especially with how fast time seems to fly by these days. Our souls, on the other hand, will last for all of eternity. Mind, body, and spirit – all three go hand in hand. When one suffers, the entire person suffers.

If you do not currently pray with your kiddos or bring them to Mass, I highly encourage you to start. If you don't know where to go, google Catholic churches near you. And if no one has ever invited you – consider this your invitation!

My husband and I were raised Catholic, and we choose to raise our kids Catholic as well. The history of the Catholic Church goes all the way back to Jesus and the Apostles, whereas other faiths have been started by individuals (not by Christ). Don't get me wrong, the Catholic Church is not perfect, nor will it ever be as it is organized by humans, and humans are born with original sin and are not perfect (besides Mary and Jesus). But how can Jesus' Church get better? You and me. The way we raise our kids, the next generation. I want to help Jesus' Church, not run from it – for my children's sake and for our world's sake.

Mind, body, and spirit. I truly believe that each of these tactics, tricks, or whatever we want to call them, are each making a small difference in the overall health of my four babies. And I pray that my three girls don't have to suffer as much, or at all, with PCOS or other reproductive diseases as a result.

Chapter 7

FINAL THOUGHTS AND RESOURCES
TO CONSIDER

If you or someone you know is suffering with PCOS or other female reproductive diseases, know that I understand your struggles. Don't give up. Thankfully there is a growing awareness of the disease and many support groups you can belong to. And remember – you are your #1 advocate (not doctors, not family, not the government – YOU!) Following is a list of people and resources that have been helpful to me during my research and journey that you may want to consider.

Something else that might help – the last pages of this book include a simple planning framework where you can create a timeline if you choose to attempt any of the ideas shared in chapter four. As a teacher, I'm very good at breaking down large problems into smaller, more doable steps that can lead to more successful outcomes. Take a look at those pages and jot somethings down as a starting point.

I am beyond grateful for having found the Creighton Model FertilityCare system and Low Dose Naltrexone, especially. I pray this book has given you motivation to be a self-advocate as well as added perspective and knowledge you may need to get the help that you and your loved ones deserve. Above all, remember this – God created you, He loves you, and He wants you to be happy and healthy to enjoy the gift of life to the fullest. Prayers, peace, joy, and everything good from me to you in your life's journey.

- PCOS Living (pcosliving.com)

- PCOS Nutrition Center (pcosnutrition.com)

- NFP (Natural Family Planning) Fertility Charting (Creighton Model charting app for Apple devices)

- Creighton Model Fertility Care System (creightonmodel.com)

- My Catholic Doctor (mycatholicdoctor.com)

- St. Gianna's Center for Women's Health and Fertility Care (stgiannacenter.com)

- Low Dose Naltrexone Research Trust (ldnresearchtrust.org)

- AgelessRx online pharmacy where LDN can be prescribed (www.agelessrx.com)

- The Healthy Choice Pharmacy (Look them up on YouTube)

- Dr. Mindy Pelz (lots of YouTube videos on hormones, women's health, menopause, and more)

- Dr. Sten Ekberg (lots of YouTube videos on overall health)

- Dr. Nicole Apelian's and Claude Davis' *The Lost Book of Herbal Remedies*

- Female Saints who can help with hardships we face as women:
    - **St. Rita** (Patroness for impossible causes, especially for sterility, abuse victims, loneliness, marriage difficulties, parenthood, widows, and disease – various miracles have been attributed to her intercession)
    - **St. Joan of Arc** (Patroness of France – pray to her for perseverance and courage)
    - **St. Opportuna of Montreuil** (Helping couples get pregnant)
    - **St. Gerard Majella** (Patron Saint of motherhood)
    - **St. Gianna Beretta Molla** (Patroness Saint of infertility, fertility, pregnant women, and mothers)
    - **Our Blessed Mother, Mary!**

I *WILL* Conquer This Disease!
How I Plan to Get Started...

What strategies / ideas / topics spoke to you the most in this book?

Creighton Model	Limiting Coffee	Sugar is Poison!	H2O	Chronobiology
Low Dose Naltrexone	Lemon Balm & Spearmint	Berries	Supplements	Exercise
Intermittent Fasting	Vitamin D	Hydroponic Gardening	Sleep	Magnesium
Full Body Massages	Garlic	Heat Therapy		

Remember – it can take up to three months for women to notice changes in their hormones. *Patience is a virtue!* Use this chart or make a similar one to create a plan and timeline for yourself to help you succeed in   your journey:

Creighton Model FertilityCare System –
Tracking my cervical mucus?

What Do I Need?	When Will I Start?	Notes/Observations

Low Dose Naltrexone Prescription?

What Do I Need?	When Will I Start?	Notes/Observations

Intermittent Fasting?

What Do I Need?	When Will I Start?	Notes/Observations

Limiting Coffee?

What Do I Need?	When Will I Start?	Notes/Observations

Lemon Balm & Spearmint?

What Do I Need?	When Will I Start?	Notes/Observations

Vitamin D – Getting More Sunshine?

What Do I Need?	When Will I Start?	Notes/Observations

Sugar Is Poison! – Replacing Processed Sugars with Healthy, Natural Sugars/Sweeteners

What Do I Need?	When Will I Start?	Notes/Observations

Berries – Grow My Own, Buy More, Eat More?

What Do I Need?	When Will I Start?	Notes/Observations

Hydroponic Gardening – Grow My Own Healthy Greens Inside My House All Year Long!

What Do I Need?	When Will I Start?	Notes/Observations

H2O – Drink More (No artificial sweeteners!)

What Do I Need?	When Will I Start?	Notes/Observations

Supplements – Maybe Amare and/or Nutritional Yeast?

What Do I Need?	When Will I Start?	Notes/Observations

Sleep – Go to Bed Earlier, Try an Amare Supplement, Banana Tea?

What Do I Need?	When Will I Start?	Notes/Observations

Chronobiology – Blue Screen Glasses?

What Do I Need?	When Will I Start?	Notes/Observations

Exercise – Go to the Gym, Take Classes, Daily Planks at Home, Walk Outside?

What Do I Need?	When Will I Start?	Notes/Observations

Magnesium – Spray, Epsom Salt Baths, Diet, Supplementing, Banana Tea?

What Do I Need?	When Will I Start?	Notes/Observations

Full Body Massage – Massage Therapist or Ashley Black Fascia Blaster Device to Use in the Shower?

What Do I Need?	When Will I Start?	Notes/Observations

Garlic – For cooking, Fermenting in Honey, Garlic Oil?

What Do I Need?	When Will I Start?	Notes/Observations

Heat Therapy _______________________

What Do I Need?	When Will I Start?	Notes/Observations

Other _______________________

What Do I Need?	When Will I Start?	Notes/Observations